TABLE OF CONTENTS

PREFACE	3
HOW TO USE THIS BOOK	5
NIPPLE DISCHARGE AND PAPILLOMA	7
MASTITIS, ABSCESS, AND INFLAMMATORY BREAST CANCER	13
BENIGN AND HIGH RISK BREAST	20
LOBULAR CARCINOMA IN SITU	26
DUCTAL CARCINOMA IN SITU	30
EARLY BREAST CANCER, CLINICALLY NODE NEGATIVE	35
LARGER AND LOCALLY ADVANCED BREAST CANCERS	41
BREAST CANCER IN PREGNANCY AND YOUNG WOMEN	47
MALE BREAST	53
ANGIOSARCOMA OF THE BREAST	58
ABOUT THE AUTHORS	62
ADDITIONAL REVIEW RESOURCES	64

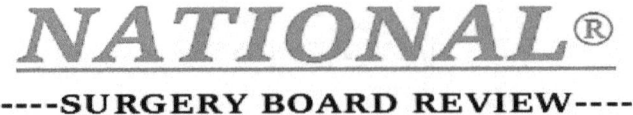
----SURGERY BOARD REVIEW----

We offer a wide range of preparatory materials and courses including:

Written Examination Board Review Course

ABSITE Preparatory Online Review Course

Mock Oral Review & Preparation Course

Oral Examination Review Manuals

Board Review Roundtable Webcast

Individual Preparatory Mock Oral Sessions

WWW.NATIONALSURGERYREVIEW.COM
1-844-REVIEW-1

Text "nationalsurgery" to 41411 for more information

2017-© National Surgery Board Review

PREFACE

The certifying examination of the American Board of Surgery is the culmination of a long road of testing and academic accomplishments that for many surgeons spans as long as two decades of higher education. The successful passage of this test earns surgeons the "seal of approval" that demonstrates to the public their competence as a surgeon caring for the community they serve. It also serves as validation to them that they have accomplished a level of proficiency and ability that they have so diligently worked for throughout decades of higher education and surgical training.

The format of this exam, however, is very different from the far more familiar written exams that students become accustomed to throughout college and medical school. Its nature can evoke a great amount of anxiety, and the mystique and urban legends associated with it are familiar to surgical trainees everywhere in the United States. The test is also seen as a right of passage and proof of the ability to not only master the broad knowledge base of surgical principles but also of the ability to think through the toughest and most difficult of surgical situations.

The very first task in the establishment of our surgery board review platform was to contact the American Board of Surgery and discuss the ethics and nuances of running a board review institute. It is clear that this exam requires more than knowledge, and besides, knowledge is already tested on the qualifying exam. The purpose of the certifying exam is to demonstrate that one can reason and safely apply the knowledge demonstrated on the qualifying exam in a typical surgical practice.

Our scope is to review those everyday common scenarios and help candidates deliver the answers based on the knowledge they already possess in an efficient

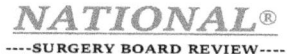

and organized manner. We will never review topics taken straight from previous exams, but our commonly encountered scenarios may overlap with those that the Board of Surgery expects its diplomats to master. It is not practical to think that anyone could mislead the examiners into believing that they are safe when in reality they may not be. The examiners are accomplished surgical educators and much too sophisticated. They can easily identify a candidate who may be book smart but lacking the capabilities to practically apply that knowledge. But proficient physicians who are quite adept may stumble on topics which they treat on a daily basis without proper preparation and re-enforcement of common concepts.

Board review courses hold an important role in recapitulating the pearls and principles of surgery. Our goal is to review those details and help the candidates deliver their answers in a way that demonstrates the sharpness of their knowledge and their reasoning capabilities. Some argue that our courses, lectures and review materials give candidates an advantage in the course of the examination. We agree; *that is what good preparation is supposed to do.*

~ Adrian G. Dan, MD FACS
Founder, National Surgery Board Review

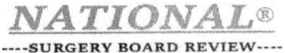

HOW TO USE THIS BOOK

- **This text is not intended to replace or be used in lieu of a complete surgical reference textbook in the clinical management of general surgery patients.**

- These scenarios are written to assist candidates in preparing for the certifying oral examination of the American Board of Surgery. Our intent is not to duplicate any questions that have been previously asked in the examination, but to ethically review commonly encountered scenarios in the practice of general surgery. The review of such scenarios is important in order to formulate, organize and deliver the answers that demonstrate an ample understanding of the safe and sound practice of surgery.

- The scenarios are not meant to be a complete comprehensive review of the specific topic, but one particular pathway in the infinite myriad of potential pathways along which a case may progress. Not all knowledge related to each topic is covered and not all possible questions are asked in the book or on the certifying exam for that matter. It would not be feasible or practical to review all potential pathways as would be the role of a comprehensive surgical textbook. Likewise, the answers are meant to review commonly utilized therapies that are considered standard of care. These answers are by no means *"the best" or "the only"* safe options but represent one commonly accepted way to manage a specific condition. <u>The scenarios are limited by design to efficiently cover the most important concepts in each particular topic.</u>

- Each review book is designed to quickly and efficiently review the designated topic. It is beyond the scope of any specific section to review all the principles of

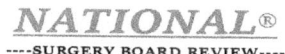

general surgery. For that reason you may be redirected from time to time to another booklet within the NATIONAL® Surgery Board Review series. For example, a particular complication may potentially occur within many different pathways (e.g. anastomotic leak). The management of this complication may not be covered in full depth in every single scenario for the sake of efficiency. However it may be covered in great detail in the *Surgical Complications* booklet. Similarly a particular procedure (e.g. bowel anastomosis) may be described in full detail in one of the *Common Surgical Procedures* booklets of the series.

- The responses to the questions in this book are carefully thought out and edited with the help of experts and reference material. Do not let the fact that your own answer may be slightly different break your confidence. There are indeed other safe ways to manage a condition in addition to the listed answer, and the review will add to what you should already know. You are not expected to recite a list of responses as if it were read from a textbook. The examiners are not trying to assess your ability to memorize but your ability to reason. Therefore, do not feel intimidated when reading the answers and understand that a safe and reasonable answer is what is expected of you on the oral examination.

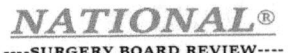

1. NIPPLE DISCHARGE AND PAPILLOMA

PATIENT PRESENTATION:

A 55-year-old woman presents to the office with complaint of nipple discharge. She has no medical problems, and denies any other breast symptoms. Her last mammogram was 6 months ago and was normal.

QUESTION / ANSWER DIALOGUE:

- What additional questions would you ask specifically about the nipple discharge?

  Important questions to ask about nipple discharge include duration of symptoms; frequency (daily or only occurred once); color of the discharge; multiple or single ducts; bilateral or unilateral; spontaneous or with manipulation. These questions help you to understand whether this is more likely physiologic or pathologic discharge. Qualities of physiologic discharge include white/yellow/green discoloration, from multiple ducts, bilateral discharge, and present with manipulation. Qualities of pathologic discharge include bloody or clear color, one duct, unilateral, and spontaneous expression.

- The patient describes to you what sounds like physiologic discharge. On physical exam you are able to express white discharge from multiple ducts bilaterally. What do you advise the patient?

  You can reassure the patient that it appears to be physiologic discharge. However, there are some laboratory evaluations that should be ordered to ensure there is no underlying medical issue. Prolactin levels and thyroid function testing would be appropriate.

If lab results are normal, it is safe to see the patient back in 3-6 months for re-check of symptoms. She should be instructed to call or return sooner if pathologic discharge features develop. If upon return visit she remains with physiologic discharge and normal labs, no additional work-up is required, and she can return to yearly clinical breast examinations and yearly screening mammograms.

- The patient describes to you what sounds like pathologic discharge. On physical examination, you note bloody discharge from a single duct on the right side. How would you proceed with work-up?

The initial imaging evaluation should include unilateral diagnostic mammogram (including spot compression of the retro-areolar region), along with ultrasound examination looking for a retroareolar mass or papilloma. Even if the patient had a screening mammogram within the past year, a new symptom warrants a new mammogram. Screening mammograms are routine mammograms recommended for all women yearly starting at the age of 40. Diagnostic mammograms are for women who report a problem (mass, nipple discharge, or have an abnormal screening mammogram).

Papillomas are often described as an intra-ductal mass with associated ductal dilation, with or without calcifications. All masses visualized on imaging work-up for bloody nipple discharge should have an image-guided biopsy for tissue diagnosis.

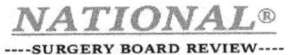

While ductograms are often referenced to work-up pathologic nipple discharge, in practice they can be difficult to perform and often have low yield. It is not wrong to perform a ductogram as an additional step in the work-up, but this should be after a diagnostic mammogram and an ultrasound. MRI is another imaging tool that can be used for evaluation of bloody nipple discharge if other imaging modalities are negative and suspicion is high. This should be considered only after a diagnostic mammogram and ultrasound.

- The patient's diagnostic mammogram is normal. Her ultrasound demonstrates a 0.5cm irregular intra-ductal mass with angular margins and associated ductal dilation. Ultrasound guided core biopsy is performed. Pathology confirms the diagnosis of papilloma with atypia. What do you recommend and why?

  Wire-localized excisional biopsy should be performed. Papilloma with atypia is associated with up to 25-30% rate of upgrade to DCIS or invasive cancer when the complete area is excised in the operating room.

- Instead of the above, the patient's diagnostic mammogram, ultrasound, and MRI demonstrate no abnormalities. She continues to have bloody nipple discharge from a single duct. What do you recommend and why?

  Duct excision should be performed. Despite normal imaging, the patient continues to have pathologic nipple discharge, so this operation is warranted to ensure there is no imaging-occult abnormality (such as papilloma or DCIS) causing her symptoms. To perform this operation, a lacrimal probe is inserted into the duct with the abnormal discharge. Dissection is carefully carried out from the base of the nipple around the abnormal duct (getting a small rim of normal breast tissue) for a length of about 2-3cm. Alternatively, a central duct excision can be performed.

KEY TEACHING POINTS:

NIPPLE DISCHARGE AND PAPILLOMA

- The most important part of evaluation for nipple discharge is to ask appropriate questions to understand whether it is pathologic or physiologic discharge, since the work-up and treatment varies significantly, as was described in the clinical vignettes above.

- The standard imaging work-up for any breast abnormality or symptom includes diagnostic mammogram and ultrasound. Image guided biopsy is always the preferred method for obtaining tissue for a diagnosis. If the patient's abnormality is seen by mammogram only (such as asymmetry or calcifications), stereotactic biopsy is recommended. If the patient's abnormality is seen by ultrasound (such as mass), then ultrasound guided biopsy is preferred.

- Papilloma is the most common cause of bloody nipple discharge. A papilloma itself is NOT cancer, but if there is atypia on the biopsy, there is up to a 25-30% chance of cancer upon excision. Thus excisional biopsy is recommended for the lesions.

- In certain cases, a papilloma WITHOUT atypia can be monitored rather than excised. If the patient's imaging and pathology are concordant; if the papilloma is small without atypia (essentially an incidental finding); if there is no associated mass; and if the patient is asymptomatic, close clinical and imaging follow-up can be considered instead of operative excision. However, when in doubt, wire localized excision of the papilloma is a safe answer.

REFERENCES:

Nakhlis F, et al. Papilloma on core biopsy: Excision vs. observation. *Ann Surg Onc.* 2015;22:1479-82.

Pareja F, et al. Breast intraductal papillomas without atypia in radiologic-pathologic concordant core-needle biopsies: Rate of upgrade to carcinoma at excision. Cancer 2016;122:2819-27.

Townsend CM, et al. Editors. Sabiston Textbook of Surgery 20th Ed. Philadelphia, PA: Elsevier; 2016.

NOTES:

2. MASTITIS, ABSCESS, AND INFLAMMATORY BREAST CANCER

PATIENT PRESENTATION:

A 40-year-old woman presents to your clinic with an uncomfortable red and swollen right breast for the last week. She has never had problems with the breast before.

QUESTION / ANSWER DIALOGUE:

- What must you consider in your differential diagnosis? What additional history questions or findings on examination would make you consider one differential over another?

    - *Mastitis – Generalized swelling and erythema of the breast due to infection. Patients who are breast feeding or diabetic are more prone to mastitis compared to other patients. Often on examination there is tenderness and warmth of the breast with blanching erythema.*

    - *Abscess – More localized process of swelling and erythema. Abscess can develop in the setting of mastitis as well. Patients who are breast feeding, diabetic, and smokers may be more prone to abscesses compared to other individuals. On examination, you may feel a distinct area of fluctuance, induration, or other evidence of underlying fluid collection. Particularly in larger-breasted women, a deeper abscess can be sometimes difficult to feel on examination, so ultrasound can be useful.*

- - Inflammatory breast cancer – Inflammatory cancer should be in the differential diagnosis for any patient with erythema of the breast. Often the erythema is more gradual onset than with mastitis or abscess, but it can progress quickly in some cases. Inflammatory breast cancer is a clinical diagnosis; at least 1/3 of the breast to be erythematous to meet the diagnostic criteria. Peau d'orange appearance with or without associated mass are common but not required for diagnosis.

- You think the patient has mastitis based on your history and examination. What do you recommend for further evaluation and treatment?

Mastitis is treated with oral antibiotics, which cover skin flora such as penicillin. If a patient has a history of MRSA infection, Bactrim may be reasonable. You should see the patient back in one week, sooner if symptoms or erythema worsen. If the area is improving, patients should complete the course of antibiotics and be seen back to ensure complete resolution. If the area is minimally improved or stable, you can try changing the antibiotics and again re-evaluating in a week to see how she is doing. Ultrasound can be considered to rule out underlying abscess. Mammograms are not routinely performed for acute mastitis, but you can use ultrasound to ensure there is no underlying abscess. Patients can safely continue to pump or breast feed during mastitis. Diabetic patients can be referred to endocrinology for help with blood sugar control.

- You think the patient has an abscess based on the history and examination. What do you recommend for further evaluation and treatment?

    Ultrasound-guided aspiration of the abscess is the first preferred step over incision and drainage, particularly if it is located deeper inside the breast, if the patient is breast-feeding, and/or if it appears simple (without loculations). Patients should be warned that often multiple aspirations (2-3) are required for complete resolution. Fluid aspirated should be sent for culture, and the patient should be started on oral antibiotics. You should see the patient back in one week, sooner if her symptoms are progressing, for repeat examination, imaging and aspiration. If the abscess is complex or very large, then I&D may be performed with placement of packing as necessary. This can be done either at the bedside or in the OR. I&D should be avoided in lactating patients if possible due to the risk of milk fistula formation.

- The patient was initially treated for mastitis with two 14 day courses of oral antibiotics (28 days total). Her erythema is not improved. What should you consider, and how would you evaluate the patient for this?

    Close follow-up to ensure resolution is required in all patients with presumed mastitis because mastitis can mimic inflammatory breast cancer. If the patient is not getting better after antibiotic treatment, inflammatory cancer should be strongly considered, and skin punch biopsy should be performed. This is done in the office under local anesthetic. Any area of thickened and erythematous breast tissue can be skin punched and sent to pathology for review. A positive biopsy will demonstrate tumor cells invading the dermal lymphatics.

If you are concerned for inflammatory breast cancer, mammogram should be performed as most patients also have an underlying breast mass. Biopsy of either the breast mass or the erythematous skin can be diagnostic. Remember that inflammatory breast cancer is also a clinical diagnosis – so a woman with a biopsy-proven breast cancer with at least 1/3 of her breast with erythematous skin meets the clinical criteria for inflammatory breast cancer.

- The patient's skin punch biopsy returns positive for dermal lymphatic invasion (diagnostic for inflammatory breast cancer). What stage cancer does she have?

Inflammatory breast cancer is T4 disease. Many patients with inflammatory cancer also have lymph node involvement, so careful clinical and imaging examination of the patient is mandatory. A patient with inflammatory breast cancer automatically has clinical stage III disease (T4, N0-3).

- What is the treatment for inflammatory breast cancer?

For all patients with inflammatory breast cancer, the treatment sequence is ALWAYS neoadjuvant chemotherapy followed by surgery and then radiation. Surgery must always be modified radical mastectomy for any patient with inflammatory breast cancer. You should never do only a sentinel lymph node biopsy for these patients, nor are the patients candidates for lumpectomy or skin- or nipple-sparing mastectomy.

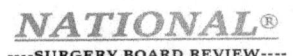

Surgery is always followed by radiation treatment. The patient may be a candidate for delayed reconstruction (after completion of radiation treatment) and disease is stable for a period of time. Recurrence rates in these patients are high.

KEY TEACHING POINTS:

MASTITIS, ABSCESS, AND INFLAMMATORY BREAST CANCER

- Infections of the breast (mastitis and/or abscess) are very common, particularly in patients who are breast-feeding and/or diabetic. Smokers also frequently get infections of the breast, which can be chronic in nature and quite difficult to heal completely.

- Any patient with a breast infection should be followed until resolution, and inflammatory cancer is in the differential diagnosis. Inflammatory cancer is a rare (between 2-5% of breast cancers) but very aggressive subtype. It is very important to know that inflammatory breast cancer is a clinical diagnosis supported by pathologic findings. If there is any concern for inflammatory breast cancer, skin punch biopsy should be completed, not excisional biopsy.

- Five-year survival has improved with the above documented regimen for treatment (neoadjuvant chemotherapy, modified radical mastectomy, and radiation) but remains lower than other women with similar stage non-inflammatory disease.

REFERENCES:

NCCN Clinical Practice Guidelines in Oncology, Breast Cancer NCCN Evidence Blocks. – Version 2.2016 – NCCN.org

Norton JA, et al. Editors. Surgery: Basic Science and Clinical Evidence 2nd Ed. New York, NY: Springer; 2008.

Townsend CM, et al. Editors. Sabiston Textbook of Surgery 20th Ed. Philadelphia, PA: Elsevier; 2016.

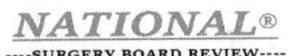

NOTES:

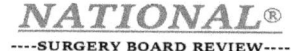

3. BENIGN AND HIGH RISK BREAST

PATIENT PRESENTATION:

A 62-year-old woman presents to outpatient clinic after an abnormal mammogram showing an asymmetry and subsequent imaging-guided biopsy. The patient has no family history or personal history of breast disease or issues. She has no symptoms.

QUESTION / ANSWER DIALOGUE:

- The biopsy results are consistent with atypical ductal hyperplasia. What additional work-up is recommended, and what do you advise the patient?

  Aside from a focused breast physical examination, no additional work-up is required. You should verify that the pathology and imaging results are concordant to make sure nothing is missed. Atypical ductal hyperplasia (ADH) is a benign but high-risk diagnosis. Wire localized excisional biopsy is recommended for these lesions as up to 15-30% of patients are upgraded to DCIS or invasive cancer upon excision. It is okay if the margins on the excisional biopsy are positive because the purpose is not to clear all disease, but rather to take out additional tissue for pathology to make sure there is no in situ or invasive cancer present. Re-excision for positive margin is not recommended.

- The biopsy results are consistent with radial scar. What additional work-up is recommended, and what do you advise the patient?

Similar to ADH, breast examination is the only additional work-up required. No additional imaging is needed. After verifying that the pathology and imaging results are concordant, wire localized excisional biopsy should be recommended as there is up to a 15% chance of upgrade to cancer at the time of excision.

- The biopsy results are consistent with pseudoangiomatous stromal hyperplasia (PASH). What additional work-up should you do, and what do you advise the patient?

  PASH is often clinically appreciated on examination as a thickening or mass-like area in the breast, and can even appear as a mass-like lesion on imaging. If you confirm that there is pathology and imaging concordance, no further treatment is required. Excisional biopsy is usually not recommended. The patient should be re-evaluated in 3 months with clinical examination, and often imaging is repeated in 6 months' time. If there is significant enlargement of the area on follow-up, excisional biopsy should be performed as enlargement of a benign area can also become concerning. Also, if there is discordance between the pathology and imaging, excisional biopsy should be recommended.

- What diagnoses (above examples or others) are considered high-risk for developing future breast cancers? What do you advise the patient about follow-up going forward? Is there anything else she should consider for treatment at this time if she has a high-risk lesion?

ADH, atypical lobular hyperplasia (ALH), and radial scar are all high-risk lesions with increased risk of developing a future breast cancer, especially if there is a family history of breast cancer. LCIS is also a high-risk lesion; management is discussed in a later chapter. These diagnoses increase the risk of developing cancer for both breasts, and thus increased surveillance of both breasts is recommended. Usually patients should get clinical breast examinations every 6 months and continue with annual mammograms. Yearly MRI (alternating with the timing of mammogram) can be considered, but MRI should NOT replace mammograms as a means of screening for breast cancer.

Chemoprevention can be offered to women who are at high risk for breast cancer to decrease this risk. This would consist of tamoxifen for pre-menopausal patients or aromatase inhibitor for post-menopausal patients. If a patient takes chemoprevention for 5 years, she reduces her risk of breast cancer by about 50%. This protective impact persists for about 10-15 years, so it continues to help the patient even after she has completed the course of her treatment. The side effects of Tamoxifen are blood clots, stroke and increased risk of endometrial cancer. The main side effect of aromatase inhibitors is osteoporosis.

Prophylactic mastectomy for high-risk but benign lesions is generally not recommended.

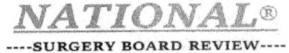

KEY TEACHING POINTS:

BENIGN AND HIGH RISK BREAST

- Some benign pathology diagnoses are considered high-risk lesions, and excisional biopsy is recommended. These include ADH, ALH, radial scar, and LCIS. Upon excisional biopsy, negative margins are NOT required. The purpose of the biopsy is to get more tissue for pathology to ensure a cancer is not being missed, not to completely remove the area. Patients with these diagnoses should be considered for chemoprevention and followed closely with clinical and imaging evaluations.

- Breast pain, breast cyst, fibrocystic change, sclerosing adenosis, fat necrosis, and fibrosis are all benign diagnoses. You should ensure that the pathology and imaging results are concordant to make sure nothing was missed. No increased follow-up is required, and excision in the operating room is not required.

- Fibroadenoma is a common, benign breast mass found in teenagers and pre-menopausal women. A fibroadenoma in the peri-menopausal or post-menopausal population is abnormal and should be considered suspicious. Fibroadenomas are often diagnosed by ultrasound evaluation, but image-guided biopsy is recommended to confirm the diagnosis, as the differential includes phyllodes tumor.

    - If on the core biopsy the pathologist cannot distinguish between fibroadenoma and phyllodes, they may diagnose the lesion as a fibroepithelial lesion – which does require excision. A phyllodes tumor is characterized by leaf-like architecture and (benign, intermediate or malignant) and should be excised with 1cm margins.

- A biopsy-proven fibroadenoma does not require excision; it can be followed with serial ultrasound every 6 months for 2 years to confirm stability. If the fibroadenoma grows by >10%, is larger than 2-2.5cm in size, or causes symptoms (pain), excision is recommended.

REFERENCES:

Norton J, et al. Editors. Surgery: Basic Science and Clinical Evidence 2nd Ed. NY, NY: Springer; 2008.

Townsend CM, et al. Editors. Sabiston Textbook of Surgery 20th Ed. Philadelphia, PA: Elsevier; 2016.

NOTES:

4. LOBULAR CARCINOMA IN SITU

PATIENT PRESENTATION:

A 58-year-old woman presents to the clinic after having a stereotactic biopsy for an asymmetry, which demonstrated lobular carcinoma in situ (LCIS). She has no breast symptoms, no personal or family history of breast disease, and is otherwise healthy.

QUESTION / ANSWER DIALOGUE:

- Does this patient have a diagnosis of breast cancer?

    No. LCIS is NOT breast cancer. It is a very high-risk lesion, which requires further management, but is not an actual diagnosis of cancer.

- What do you advise the patient for management?

    LCIS requires excisional biopsy as there is a risk of upstaging to cancer upon excision.

- What margins are required on final pathology for LCIS?

    For classic LCIS (most common), negative margins are not required. The excisional biopsy is done to get extra tissue for pathology to ensure there is no underlying malignancy, not to remove the entire area. For pleomorphic LCIS (less common), positive margins are NOT acceptable because this lesion is very difficult to distinguish from DCIS, so you should return to the OR if needed to ensure you have clear margins.

- The patient wants to have a mastectomy with a diagnosis of LCIS. Is this reasonable?

  While LCIS is not a cancer diagnosis, it does confer up to a 20-40% lifetime risk of developing breast cancer in either breast and is thus considered particularly high risk. High-risk discussion for management in these patients is appropriate. Prophylactic mastectomy for risk reduction with a diagnosis of LCIS can be considered, especially with a strong family history of breast cancer.

- The patient underwent excisional biopsy, and the final pathology was consistent with classic LCIS. What additional follow-up or treatment would you recommend?

  LCIS diagnosis puts the patient at increased risk for developing both ductal and lobular types of invasive breast cancer, with up to 2-40% risk documented lifetime in prior studies. Patients should at minimum have increased screening with twice yearly breast examinations and annual mammograms. MRI yearly (alternating with mammogram) can be offered; this does NOT replace mammogram screening but can be used as an adjunct in high-risk patients, such as those with LCIS. Chemoprevention with tamoxifen (pre-menopausal) or aromatase inhibitors (post-menopausal) for five years decreases future risk of breast cancer by about 50%, and is reasonable to recommend to these patients. Prophylactic bilateral mastectomy can also be considered.

KEY TEACHING POINTS:

LOBULAR CARCINOMA IN SITU

- Do not confuse LCIS with DCIS! Lobular carcinoma in situ (LCIS) is NOT a diagnosis of breast cancer and thus should NOT be treated with chemotherapy or radiation. Ductal carcinoma in situ (DCIS) is a diagnosis of breast cancer (Stage 0 cancer by definition). Chemotherapy is not recommended for DCIS since it is in situ disease; radiation is recommended for women with DCIS who undergo partial mastectomy. Both patients with LCIS and DCIS commonly receive Tamoxifen or aromatase inhibitors to decrease the risk of developing a new cancer or decrease risk for disease recurrence.

- There are two types of LCIS: classic and pleomorphic. Both require excisional biopsy. A positive margin on classic LCIS excision is fine; there is no need to return to the OR to clear the margins. A positive margin on pleomorphic LCIS is not okay (pleomorphic LCIS appears very similar to DCIS), and the patient should return to the OR to ensure clear margins. Radiation is not needed for pleomorphic LCIS, only clear margins.

- MRI screening as a tool for high-risk screening is recommended in women with a calculated estimated lifetime risk of breast cancer >20%. General guidelines for when an annual MRI is recommended include known genetic BRCA mutation (start MRI at age 25); 1st degree relative with positive genetic mutation and patient untested (start MRI at age 25); and lifetime risk of breast cancer >20% by risk calculation models. In addition, patients with history of chest radiation (such as for lymphoma) or high-risk lesions (such as LCIS) are

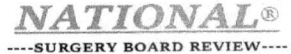

reasonable candidates for MRI screening. Annual MRI does not replace annual mammogram screening, but rather is an adjunct for mammograms.

REFERENCES:

NCCN Clinical Practice Guidelines in Oncology, Breast Cancer NCCN Evidence Blocks. – Version 2.2016 – NCCN.org

Townsend CM, et al. Editors. Sabiston Textbook of Surgery 20th Ed. Philadelphia, PA: Elsevier; 2016.

NOTES:

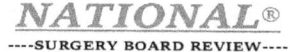

5. DUCTAL CARCINOMA IN SITU

PATIENT PRESENTATION:

A 45-year-old woman presents to the office after a stereotactic biopsy of new calcifications in her right breast. Biopsy demonstrates ductal carcinoma in situ (DCIS).

QUESTION / ANSWER DIALOGUE:

- Describe DCIS in terms of pathology findings.

    DCIS by definition is in situ disease, which means that the breast cancer cells are filling up the ducts of the breast, but there is no evidence yet that the cancer cells have invaded the basement membrane and gone outside of the ducts into the surrounding breast tissue.

- What imaging findings are important to review in patients with a diagnosis of DCIS?

    DCIS can present as a mass or asymmetry, but most often presents as calcifications on imaging. It is important to understand the extent of disease on imaging. Often the calcifications extend for several centimeters from the area of the biopsy or are present in multiple areas around the breast. If there is concern for additional areas of DCIS or extent of disease, additional image-guided biopsies can be recommended to confirm extent or multi-focality.

- What surgical options would you offer to a patient with DCIS?

For the surgical treatment for DCIS there are two options: lumpectomy + radiation or mastectomy.

Wire localized lumpectomy is an option for patients with a single focus of DCIS. Clear margins for 2 mm are required for DCIS. Sentinel lymph node excision is not required for lumpectomy for DCIS because by definition the cancer is confined to the ducts and has not gone outside of the ducts, including to the lymph nodes. If final pathology demonstrates invasive breast cancer (up-staged), then the patient will need to return to the OR for sentinel lymph node excision. Patients with DCIS who undergo lumpectomy also require radiation to prevent recurrence.

Simple mastectomy is also a reasonable option for patients with DCIS. This option is offered for patients even with a small area of DCIS. It is recommended for patients with extensive DCIS or patients with multiple areas of DCIS confirmed on biopsy. If you are doing a mastectomy for DCIS, it is reasonable to perform a sentinel lymph node excision at the same time. If you do not perform a sentinel lymph node excision at the time of mastectomy and the final pathology reports invasive cancer (up-staged), then the patient would need to have an axillary dissection for lymph node evaluation, as you are no longer able to map for sentinel lymph node excision. Radiation treatment is not required for patients with DCIS who undergo mastectomy.

- What is the difference between multifocal and multicentric disease?

Multifocal disease (DCIS or invasive cancer) is more than 1 foci of disease located in the same quadrant of the breast. Multicentric disease is more than 1 foci of disease located in different quadrants. Lumpectomy can be performed for multifocal disease, but multicentric disease requires a mastectomy.

- What tumor markers/receptors should be sent for patients with DCIS?

    Estrogen receptor (ER) and progesterone receptor (PR) should be sent for patients with DCIS. Patients with DCIS who are ER positive will be recommended to take anti-hormonal medications. HER2 is not checked for DCIS (only for invasive cancers).

KEY TEACHING POINTS:

DUCTAL CARCINOMA IN SITU

- Ductal carcinoma in situ (DCIS) is a non-invasive breast cancer (Stage 0), which requires multi-modality treatment. If left untreated, DCIS progresses to invasive cancer in about 50% of women with this diagnosis. It is unclear which women will progress to develop invasive cancer, so at this time all women with DCIS are treated for stage 0 breast cancer.

- DCIS requires surgical excision with negative margins. Recent consensus statements suggest 2mm as minimum margins for DCIS excision and is a safe answer for the boards and for practice.

- Patients may select lumpectomy or mastectomy for a diagnosis of DCIS. It is most important to understand the extent of the disease because these lesions can be extensive or multifocal. Operative management has been described above.

- Patients who have lumpectomy should be recommended to receive adjuvant radiation treatment. There is no role for chemotherapy for DCIS, even if it is high-grade or ER negative. Anti-hormonal medication is recommended for 5-10 years in ER positive patients.

REFERENCES:

NCCN Clinical Practice Guidelines in Oncology, Breast Cancer NCCN Evidence Blocks. – Version 2.2016 – NCCN.org

Townsend CM, et al. Editors. Sabiston Textbook of Surgery 20th Ed. Philadelphia, PA: Elsevier; 2016.

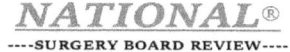

NOTES:

6. EARLY BREAST CANCER, CLINICALLY NODE NEGATIVE

PATIENT PRESENTATION:

A 65-year-old woman presents to your office with a newly diagnosed right-sided breast cancer, which was found on her screening mammogram. It is an invasive lobular carcinoma, ER+, PR+, HER2-. By imaging it is 1.2cm in size.

QUESTION / ANSWER DIALOGUE:

- Describe what you would look for on physical breast examination.

    The patient should be examined in the upright and supine positions. You should evaluate for any skin changes, nipple retraction, nipple discharge, or masses. You should check for axillary, supraclavicular, and cervical lymphadenopathy. Make sure to examine both sides, not just the side with the cancer.

- On your examination, there is no lymphadenopathy. The patient has no significant medical, surgical, or family history. What breast operation(s) would you consider for this patient?

    For the surgical treatment of breast cancer there are two options: lumpectomy + radiation or mastectomy.

    For a patent with a small breast cancer without lymphadenopathy, surgery is the first step in management. A patient is an appropriate candidate for a lumpectomy if their breast will not have significant disfigurement after excision of the tumor. To judge this, consider the tumor size (what you would have to excise) to breast size ratio. Remember if a patient chooses lumpectomy, this is always followed by radiation.

Any patient may choose mastectomy. Indications for mastectomy include multifocal disease, large tumor compared to breast size, prior history of breast cancer with radiation or other chest wall radiation. A patient cannot receive radiation twice, so if they have already had a lumpectomy with radiation and now have a recurrence or new cancer, they should have a mastectomy. Patients who are pregnant or have a skin condition, such as lupus or scleroderma, cannot have radiation and should have a mastectomy. If a patient chooses mastectomy, consultation to plastic surgery for reconstruction should always be offered.

- What lymph node operation will you recommend for this patient, and how do you perform it?

The sentinel lymph node procedure selectively identifies the first lymph node(s) draining the breast and therefore the first nodes that cancer would potentially spread to. Sentinel lymph node excision is acceptable for any clinically node-negative patient. Most sentinel lymph node operations are done with dual mapping using both radionucleotide and blue dye. Either methylene blue (side effect of skin necrosis) or isosulfan blue (side effect of anaphylaxis) can be used. Inject either peri-areolar region or peri-tumoral and massage for 5 minutes to allow the dye to go to the lymph nodes. Make a 2-3cm incision about 2 finger breaths below the hair-bearing area of the axilla and dissect through the clavipectoral fascia to get into the axillary lymph node basin. You should remove all nodes that are hot (within 10% of the highest number on the neoprobe) and/or blue. Usually this is 1-3 nodes.

- When you are in the operation room, there is no mapping for your sentinel lymph node. You cannot find any radioactive or blue lymph nodes. What do you do?

Axillary dissection is required.

- You find 2 sentinel lymph nodes with your mapping and send these for frozen evaluation. One comes back positive for cancer, the other one is negative. What do you do?

If you are doing a lumpectomy and you have only 1 or 2 sentinel nodes that are positive, no additional surgery is required. The patient will have radiation after surgery because they are having a lumpectomy, so the radiation will cover the lymph nodes.

If you are doing a mastectomy and any sentinel lymph nodes are positive OR if you are doing a lumpectomy and 3 or more sentinel lymph nodes are positive, the safe answer is to perform an axillary dissection.

- You performed a lumpectomy and on your final pathology, one of the margins is positive for cancer. What do you do?

For an invasive cancer (ductal or lobular), the recommended clear margin is "no ink on tumor". (remember a clear margin for DCIS is 2mm). Taking the patient back to the OR for margin re-excision is appropriate. Alternatively, the patient may opt for mastectomy instead of margin re-excision. You should not leave a positive margin alone. Radiation does not take care of a positive margin.

If a second trip to the operation room also results in a positive margin or if there are multiple positive margins after the first operation, mastectomy is often recommended. The exact practice in terms of number of re-excisions and number of positive margins before recommending mastectomy varies from one provider to another. These are general guidelines for safe answers for the boards.

KEY TEACHING POINTS:

EARLY BREAST CANCER, CLINICALLY NODE NEGATIVE

- For all breast cancers, make sure to identify the size of the tumor (determine T stage) and any clinical or imaging evidence of axillary lymph node involvement (N stage). Make sure both breasts have been evaluated with mammogram, not just one. It is important to ask about skin changes for all breast cancer patients as inflammatory cancer is treated differently.

- For T1 breast cancers (<2cm in size) without imaging or clinical indication of lymph node involvement, surgery is the first choice. You should know how to perform a sentinel lymph node operation, including the potential operative circumstances that could arise (non-mapping and frozen section results) and how to handle these. Patients with clinically positive lymph nodes are NOT candidates for sentinel lymph node operations.

- Remember breast cancer requires multidisciplinary care. Refer patients to radiation oncology if they have a lumpectomy or if they have any lymph node involvement. Refer all patients to medical oncology. Herceptin is the targeted therapy for HER2+ patients. ER negative cancers require chemotherapy. Many patients with lymph node involvement and/or larger tumors will get chemotherapy. For patients with node negative, ER+, HER2- small breast cancers, it can be hard to determine if they would benefit from chemotherapy or not, so Oncotype Dx testing should be recommended. This test is ordered after surgery to test tumor genes and determine if a patient is low (score <18), intermediate (score 18-30), or high risk (score >30) for disease recurrence, thus informing chemotherapy decision.

- Anti-hormonal treatment is appropriate for all patients with ER+ cancers. Tamoxifen is generally given to pre-menopausal women and aromatase inhibitors to post-menopausal women.

REFERENCES:

Fischer JE. Fischer's Mastery of Surgery 6th Ed. Philadelphia, PA: Lippincott Williams & Wilkins; 2012.

Townsend CM, et al. Editors. Sabiston Textbook of Surgery 20th Ed. Philadelphia, PA: Elsevier; 2016.

NOTES:

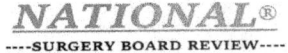

7. LARGER AND LOCALLY ADVANCED BREAST CANCERS

PATIENT PRESENTATION:

A 60-year-old woman presents to the office with a newly diagnosed right-sided breast cancer. It is palpable and 6cm in size by imaging. Biopsy was consistent with invasive ductal carcinoma.

QUESTION / ANSWER DIALOGUE:

- What are important physical breast examination considerations, particularly for larger tumors?

  Make sure to check everyone for axillary lymphadenopathy; bigger tumors have a greater chance of having lymph node involvement. Check to see if the breast is still mobile compared to the chest wall. If it is fixed or not mobile, be concerned for muscle involvement. Also make sure there is no skin or nipple involvement. MRI can be ordered to better evaluate for these findings.

- On examination, your patient has significant right-sided axillary lymphadenopathy. The breast is mobile (not fixed to the chest wall). Would you recommend any further evaluation for the axillary lymphadenopathy?

  Ultrasound guided lymph node biopsy can be considered in patients who are clinically node positive to confirm the presence of cancer in the lymph nodes before any surgery or medical treatment, if it would change your management. Lymph node positivity is considered a reasonable indication for neoadjuvant chemotherapy, especially in ER negative or HER2 amplified cancers. Patients with clinically positive lymph nodes are NOT candidates for sentinel lymph node excision and must undergo axillary dissection if you are proceeding directly to the OR rather than referring for neoadjuvant chemotherapy.

- What patients might you consider for neoadjuvant chemotherapy?

   Neoadjuvant chemotherapy can be considered for patients with larger tumors (T2 or greater), clinically or biopsy-proven lymph node involvement, triple negative status, and larger (T2 or greater) HER2 positive cancers. In small HER2 positive cancers (<2cm), surgery first is fine (neoadjuvant chemotherapy is not required). In patients where lumpectomy may not be an option due to larger tumors to breast ratio, neoadjuvant chemotherapy may be used to shrink the tumor and hopefully allow for better chance at lumpectomy. Medical oncology consultation is appropriate if you think the patient may need neoadjuvant chemotherapy.

- Your patient was referred to medical oncology but wishes to proceed with surgery first regardless of recommendations. What operation would you perform?

   Modified radical mastectomy is appropriate since the patient has a large tumor to breast ratio and biopsy positive lymph node involvement. This operation is a mastectomy + level I & II axillary lymph node dissection.

- Describe the anatomic boundaries of a simple mastectomy and axillary dissection for breast cancer. What nerves can be potentially injured with an axillary dissection?

  Simple mastectomy is completed usually through an elliptical incision, which removes the nipple areola complex and all the breast tissue. The boundaries include clavicle (superior), lateral border of the sternum (medial), inframammary fold (inferior), mid axillary line/ latissimus dorsi (lateral), and pectoralis major fascia (deep). The pectoralis major fascia, but not the muscle, should be removed as part of the mastectomy specimen.

  Axillary dissection for breast cancer involves removing level I and II lymph nodes. The boundaries for the axillary dissection include axillary vein (superior), under pec minor (medial), latissimus dorsi (laterally), and subscapularis muscle (posterior). The long thoracic motor nerve runs along the chest wall and innervates the serratus anterior; injury causes winged scapula. The thoracodorsal bundle (nerve/artery/vein) runs in the middle of the deep space of the axilla, parallel to the chest wall and the long thoracic nerve. The thoracodorsal motor nerve innervates the latissimus dorsi; injury causes arm adduction weakness. The intercostal brachial sensory nerve runs perpendicular to the chest wall across the axilla; cutting this will result in numbness to the upper inner arm.

- What do you tell the patient about risk of lymphedema after surgery?

The lifetime risk of lymphedema is 2-5% after sentinel lymph node excision and 10-20% after axillary dissection. Radiation increases the risk of lymphedema. All patients who undergo axillary dissection should be referred to occupational/physical therapy for evaluation. Patients should be instructed to notify their surgeon with any indication of arm swelling as early intervention for lymphedema (in the form of therapy and compression garments) is critical.

KEY TEACHING POINTS:

LARGER AND LOCALLY ADVANCED BREAST CANCERS

- Patients with locally advanced cancers may be candidates for neoadjuvant chemotherapy, and referral to medical oncology is appropriate. The patient should be re-evaluated prior to completion of neoadjuvant chemotherapy, and surgery planned for 4-6 weeks after completion of chemotherapy.

- In patients who are clinically node positive or with a lymph node biopsy confirming axillary involvement preoperatively, axillary dissection is recommended. Current studies are evaluating whether sentinel lymph node excision can be used after neoadjuvant chemotherapy in select patients, but axillary dissection remains the safe answer after neoadjuvant chemotherapy at this time. Certainly any patient with clinically positive nodes who does not receive neoadjuvant chemotherapy should have an axillary dissection (not sentinel lymph node excision).

- In general, metastatic work-up is not recommended for breast cancer patients presenting with disease confined to the breast (T1 or T2, node negative cancer). For patients with locally advanced disease (T3 and/or lymph node involvement), work-up for metastatic disease may be considered. If any patient has symptoms, metastatic work-up is appropriate. CT chest/abdomen/pelvis and bone scan or a PET scan are reasonable options for metastatic work-up.

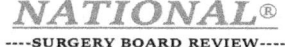

REFERENCES:

Evans SRT. Surgical Pitfalls: Prevention and Management. Philadelphia, PA: Saunders Elsevier; 2009.

NCCN Clinical Practice Guidelines in Oncology, Breast Cancer NCCN Evidence Blocks. – Version 2.2016 – NCCN.org

Norton JA, et al. Editors. Surgery: Basic Science and Clinical Evidence 2nd Ed. New York, NY: Springer; 2008.

Townsend CM, et al. Editors. Sabiston Textbook of Surgery 20th Ed. Philadelphia, PA: Elsevier; 2016.

NOTES:

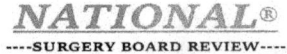

8. BREAST CANCER IN PREGNANCY AND YOUNG WOMEN

PATIENT PRESENTATION:

A 32-year-old woman who is in her second trimester of pregnancy presents to your office with concern for a new left sided breast lump. This is her first pregnancy. She has no prior breast complaints or concerns.

QUESTION / ANSWER DIALOGUE:

- What are important questions to ask regarding her symptoms?

    It is important to inquire about how long the mass has been there, if it is changing in size, any nipple discharge, any skin changes, and any associated pain/discomfort.

- Physical breast examination confirms a left sided breast mass without overlying skin changes. It is non-tender. What imaging would you order for this patient?

    Breast and axillary ultrasound is appropriate as a first step in evaluation. In addition, mammogram of BOTH breasts with shielding of the fetus is appropriate pending the results of the ultrasound. If the ultrasound demonstrates a simple cyst or an abscess, for example, mammogram may not be needed. Breast cancer must be ruled out!

- Ultrasound demonstrates an irregular 2cm mass and mammogram confirms this. There is no axillary lymphadenopathy on exam or imaging. What is your next step in evaluation?

Image guided biopsy is appropriate for all patients with concern for malignancy. Taking the patient to the operating room directly for excisional biopsy is not appropriate. You should never delay a biopsy if there is concern for breast cancer, even in a patient who is pregnant and/or breast-feeding.

- The biopsy returns as invasive ductal cancer, ER+, PR+, HER2+. By trimester, what is the preferred recommendation for management (consider surgery, chemotherapy, radiation, and hormonal therapy)?

   Radiation treatment is not administered during pregnancy.

   Hormonal therapy is not administered during pregnancy.

   Some chemotherapy (doxorubicin and cyclophosphamide) can be used in the 2nd and 3rd trimesters. Taxols and Herceptin are never administered in pregnancy due to side effects to the fetus.

   1st trimester diagnosis: Recommend modified radical mastectomy. Since the patient cannot get radiation during pregnancy, and given she still has a long time left until delivery, lumpectomy is not an appropriate surgical option for breast cancer diagnosed in the 1st trimester. Sentinel lymph node biopsy is considered risky due to the radiotracer used (blue dye may NOT be used during pregnancy) and the safe answer is to perform an axillary dissection. Chemotherapy administration should be recommended to start in the 2nd trimester.

2nd trimester diagnosis: Modified radical mastectomy OR neoadjuvant chemotherapy with operation later in 3rd trimester or after delivery. Both are appropriate options. (See next line for info about operations in the 3rd trimester).

3rd trimester: Modified radical mastectomy OR lumpectomy with radiation treatment after delivery.

KEY TEACHING POINTS:

BREAST CANCER IN PREGNANCY AND YOUNG WOMEN

- The history, examination, imaging, and image-guided biopsy for diagnosis are the same for all women with concern for breast cancer, whether or not they are pregnant. Remember to use shielding for the fetus if you are performing mammograms in pregnancy. Always order imaging of both breasts if you are concerned for breast cancer in any woman.

- The management of breast cancer in pregnancy is slightly different for each trimester. You should know the general guidelines for what can and cannot be given during pregnancy, as well as general treatment recommendations for pregnant patients with breast cancer in each trimester.

- In general for non-pregnant young women with breast cancer, the treatment is the SAME as for older women with breast cancer. They have the same options for surgery as with older women; you should not change your recommended operative intervention or other treatments based on age alone.

- Genetic testing should be offered to all young women (under the age of 50) with breast cancer. If they test positive, referral to GYN/ONC for ovarian cancer screening (CA-125 and transvaginal ultrasound every 6 months) and discussion of possible oophorectomy is appropriate given the 20-40% risk of ovarian cancer in these patients. Discussion for high-risk screening versus bilateral mastectomy given the 60-80% of breast cancer for BRCA1 or 2.

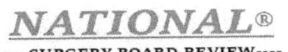

- For all breast cancer patients of any age, contralateral prophylactic mastectomy is a personal choice and is not mandatory in any patient. Any patient has the option of bilateral mastectomy if they choose. Individuals with bilateral breast cancers, those who are genetic positive, or those with a history of radiation to the chest may be more likely to benefit from bilateral mastectomy. Young age alone is not an indication for bilateral mastectomy in breast cancer.

REFERENCES:

Norton JA, et al. Editors. Surgery: Basic Science and Clinical Evidence 2nd Ed. New York, NY: Springer; 2008.

NCCN Clinical Practice Guidelines in Oncology, Breast Cancer NCCN Evidence Blocks. – Version 2.2016 – NCCN.org

Townsend CM, et al. Editors. Sabiston Textbook of Surgery 20th Ed. Philadelphia, PA: Elsevier; 2016.

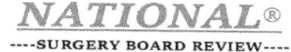

NOTES:

9. MALE BREAST

PATIENT PRESENTATION:

A 68-year-old gentleman presents to your office with a complaint of an enlarging breast mass over the past two months. He has no prior history of breast or chest wall complaints.

QUESTION / ANSWER DIALOGUE:

- What are the main differential diagnoses you need to consider?

    Gynecomastia and breast cancer.

- What are the important points to ask about in past medical history, social history and family history?

    Past medical history – Hepatic failure, kidney failure, medications (thiazides, digoxin, theophylline, androgens or other hormones), testicular mass or cancer

    Social history – Marijuana use, nutrition supplement use

    Family history – Breast or ovarian cancers, male breast cancer, pancreatic cancer, Ashkenazi ancestry

- What are the characteristics on examination that could help in your differential diagnosis?

    Gynecomastia tends to be smooth, round 2 cm prominent retroareolar tissue, often bilateral.

Breast cancer is more likely to be irregular, firm and unilateral.

- What additional work-up would you order?

    Diagnostic mammogram (bilateral) and breast ultrasound should be ordered for all patients.

    If mammogram shows a flamed shaped mass and ultrasound confirms gynecomastia, lab evaluation (LFTs, renal function testing, hormone levels) should be ordered in a focused manner based on history or examination findings.

- The patient's imaging demonstrates an irregular mass in the periphery of the breast which is concerning for cancer. How would you obtain a diagnosis?

    Image guided core biopsy is the correct answer to obtain a diagnosis for ANY patient when there is a concern for breast cancer. When you get the biopsy results, make sure to verify that the results are concordant with the imaging.

- The patient's pathology indicates an invasive ductal cancer. What additional information is needed?

    Estrogen, progesterone, and HER2 status of the tumor. Yes – even male breast cancer should be sent for estrogen and progesterone receptors! Refer all male breast cancer patients for genetic testing (they are higher risk for BRCA 2). Make sure you have examined the lymph nodes to assess for lymphadenopathy in all breast cancer patients (men and women).

- What operation is appropriate for the patient?

  Mastectomy is the operation of choice for male breast cancer patients (mainly because there is not enough tissue for a lumpectomy). But lumpectomy + radiation can be an option. Sentinel lymph node excision is appropriate if clinically node negative. Management in men is the same as women.

KEY TEACHING POINTS:

MALE BREAST

- Breast enlargement/lump in men has two main differential diagnoses: gynecomastia and breast cancer. The focus of the history, physical examination and imaging should be to distinguish between these two potential diagnoses.

- The management of gynecomastia depends on its cause. Stopping potentially causative medications or drugs, addressing underlying hormonal imbalances, or referring the patient for treatment of underlying medical problems are all appropriate. Even with these measures, gynecomastia may not regress. If you give a diagnosis of gynecomastia, it is reasonable to re-evaluate the patient with clinical breast examination in 3 months to ensure stability and that nothing has been missed. Any changes to the breast examination or patient symptoms warrant repeat imaging and clinical evaluation. Biopsy is always appropriate if the diagnosis is not straight forward on imaging.

- In men with breast cancer, all patients should be referred for genetic testing. Surgical management has already been described. If a patient is estrogen positive, he should be given tamoxifen for endocrine therapy.

REFERENCES:

Norton JA, et al. Editors. Surgery: Basic Science and Clinical Evidence 2nd Ed. New York, NY: Springer; 2008.

Townsend CM, et al. Editors. Sabiston Textbook of Surgery 20th Ed. Philadelphia, PA: Elsevier; 2016.

NOTES:

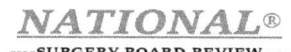

10. ANGIOSARCOMA OF THE BREAST

PATIENT PRESENTATION:

A 70-year-old woman presents to the office complaining of a one-month history of a violet/bruise colored skin lesion on her breast near her prior lumpectomy scar. She has a history of right-sided breast cancer 10 years prior, which was treated with lumpectomy and radiation.

QUESTION / ANSWER DIALOGUE:

- What should you consider on the differential diagnosis?

    New or recurrent breast cancer is always a consideration in women with a prior history of breast cancer and a new skin lesion. In a patient with a history of prior radiation, you must also consider angiosarcoma of the breast.

- Imaging is performed and does not identify any lesions within the breast, but does notice skin thickening in the area of the lesion. Skin punch biopsy is performed and confirms a diagnosis of angiosarcoma. What do you recommend for management?

    Mastectomy for wide clear margins is the recommended surgical treatment for radiation-induced angiosarcoma of the breast. These lesions are often locally aggressive, can have multifocal disease, and are difficult to manage with other forms of treatment. The local recurrence rate has been reported as high as 50% within 5 years. Axillary lymph node spread is unlikely, so routine axillary lymph node removal is not recommended. It is reasonable to perform clinical examination and ultrasound of the axilla for evaluation of any abnormal lymphadenopathy. Sometimes the amount of skin needing to be resected is extensive and a vascular flap is necessary.

- Aside from surgery, should the patient be referred for any additional treatments?

    Patients should be referred to medical oncology for consideration of chemotherapy, which may help lower the risk of recurrence. Extensive trails of chemotherapy in radiation-induced angiosarcoma are lacking due to the rarity of the disease, so medical oncology management is often variable. Referral to radiation oncology for discussion of possible treatment is also warranted, but re-radiation recommendations vary widely by provider as no good data on best approach exists. Surgery remains the mainstay of treatment for this disease.

- What is the prognosis for patients with radiation induced angiosarcoma of the breast?

    Short-term survival is often achievable (1-year survival around 90-95% has been reported) but 5-year survival is only around 50%. Very careful clinical monitoring including frequent clinical examinations is necessary as local recurrences are common. Re-excision of local recurrences with wide margins, if able, is reasonable.

KEY TEACHING POINTS:

ANGIOSARCOMA OF THE BREAST

- In patients with a history of breast cancer, including a remote history, consideration must always be given to recurrent or new breast cancer, metastatic disease, and development of secondary (radiation-induced) angiosarcoma of the breast.

- Angioscaroma is significantly more common in women with a history of radiation, but still accounts for <1% of breast cancers diagnosed in the United States each year (incidence <0.1%). The average time from radiation to angiosarcoma development is usually 10 years, with a range of 1-20 years reported in the literature.

- If diagnosis of angiosarcoma of the breast is made, these patients are best managed with aggressive surgical care, with secondary referral to medical oncology and radiation oncology for discussion of adjuvant systemic or local treatment. Axillary dissection is not required unless there is clinical or imaging evidence of disease involvement.

- It is reasonable to suggest referral to a tertiary center if a patient has a radiation-induced angiosarcoma of the breast, either for the purposes of the boards or in clinical practice.

REFERENCES:

Norton JA, et al. Editors. Surgery: Basic Science and Clinical Evidence 2nd Ed. New York, NY: Springer; 2008.

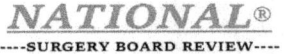

Torres KE et al. Long-term outcomes in patients with radiation-associated Angiosarcomas of the breast following surgery and radiotherapy for Breast Cancer. *Ann Surg Onc*. 2013;20(4):1267-74.

NOTES:

ABOUT THE AUTHOR

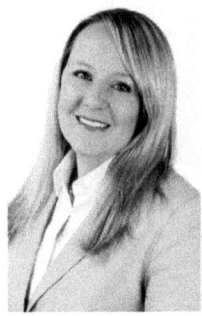

Kelsey E. Larson, MD

Dr. Larson is currently a practicing breast surgeon and faculty member at the University of Kansas She completed a breast surgical oncology fellowship at Cleveland Clinic in Cleveland OH. She received her medical degree from Case Western Reserve University and completed her General Surgery Residency training at Cleveland Clinic. She is an active member in several surgical societies and has a specific interest in clinical outcomes research, as well as resident education.

ABOUT THE AUTHOR

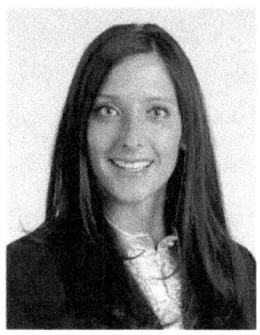

Stephanie Valente, DO

Dr. Stephanie Valente is a breast surgeon at the Cleveland Clinic and Assistant Professor of Surgery at Cleveland Clinic, Lerner College of Medicine/Case Western Reserve University in Cleveland, Ohio. Dr. Valente earned her medical degree from Ohio University, completed her surgical residency at Summa Health System, followed by a breast surgical oncology fellowship at the University of Southern California. She is certified by the American Board of Surgery in General Surgery.

Dr. Valente is the Director of the Breast Surgical Oncology fellowship program at the Cleveland Clinic and works closely with fellows, residents and medical students. Her interests include oncoplastic breast surgery, nipple sparing mastectomy, and intraoperative radiation therapy. She has authored numerous peer-reviewed journal publications and has given many presentations both nationally and internationally. She frequently directs and teaches advanced breast surgical technique training courses.

ADDITIONAL REVIEW RESOURCES

Check for upcoming:

General Surgery Written Exam Board Review Course
Comprehensive reviews of the principles of general surgery aimed to effectively prepare candidates for the in-training, qualifying and recertification exams.

ABSITE Preparatory Online Review Course
Provides a comprehensive review of the main tenants of general surgery that are commonly tested on the ABSITE.

Mock Oral Review and Preparation Course
Courses are held in the city hosting the certifying examination on the preceding weekend. Offers great preparation to help polish the delivery of answers in the oral examination format.

Oral Examination Review Manuals
Offers convenient review of topics which are commonly encountered in the practice of general surgery. These scenarios review the topics surgeons are expected to be proficient in to successfully pass the certifying oral board examination.

Board Review Roundtable Webcast
Periodic Webcasts reviewing key specific topics that are commonly encountered in practice of general surgery.

www.nationalsurgeryreview.com

1-844-REVIEW-1

Text "nationalsurgery" to 41411 for more information

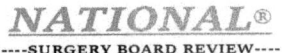

www.ingramcontent.com/pod-product-compliance
Lightning Source LLC
Chambersburg PA
CBHW061217180526
45170CB00003B/1032